Speaking

of

Alzheimer's

Julie Desmond

Speaking of Alzheimer's by Julie Desmond
Copyright © 2013 Julie Desmond
Northville, MI USA

The author and the Moore family are available to speak with your family, class or organization about our experience with Alzheimer's disease.
Inquiries to info@hospicepeople.org.

ISBN-13: 978-1493652709
ISBN-10: 1493652702

10 9 8 7 6 5 4 3 2 1

In honor of my dad, Jack I. Moore.

Dedicated to
Every family living with Alzheimer's disease
And to the people who care for them.

Protect Families.
Thanks.

Introduction: About this little book

This book will take you no time to read: twenty minutes or less… thirty if someone interrupts you while you're reading. According to the Alzheimer's Association, in America today, a person is diagnosed with Alzheimer's disease every 68 seconds. Therefore, if you are a speed reader and finish reading this book in 10 minutes, more than eight people will have been diagnosed with Alzheimer's disease during that time. If it takes you a little longer, say thirty minutes, more than twenty-six people will have received an Alzheimer's diagnosis. And if you decide to pass this book on to a friend and you chat for an hour about how things are going, you will look up to find another 53 people lined up, wearing nametags that say, "Hi! I have Alzheimer's disease!"

This book will tell you about our family, about our journey into Alzheimer's disease, and about how the Alzheimer's Association impacted our experience.

First, the facts: Alzheimer's disease is the sixth leading cause of death in the United States today, affects a third of all people over age sixty-five and costs families 17.5 billion hours in unpaid caregiving time, valued at over $215 billion – billion! – annually. And, worse, as our population ages, that number keeps growing. We're headed in the wrong direction on this thing.

Now is a good time to make a few changes on the Alzheimer's front. Right now is as good a time as any to raise awareness, drop the cultural stigma and find some effective ways to get to the end of Alzheimer's disease.

One person, one family, alone can't do much. But we can all do a little. I can write this book and you can read it and we can talk about it and then a couple more people will be thinking about this heart-breaking disease.

If you read this book and then pass it along, consider doing what my book club does with all books: write your name inside the back cover. Remember the old system of checking out library books? You could pull the tattered card out of a pocket inside the book and see the names of all the other people who have read the same book. When the topic is Alzheimer's disease, it's nice to know you are not alone; knowing someone else also read this book will help us all to remember we are in this conversation together, researching Alzheimer's disease, caring about Alzheimer's disease, living with Alzheimer's disease.

This book is not the last word on Alzheimer's. It isn't even the first word on this overwhelming topic. It is one word, one view. What you will read here began as a speech written to address a group of business people who knew little or nothing about Alzheimer's disease. It was intended to inform them through one family's first-hand account. Glean what you can, and if this book leads you to learn more about this disease, if it compels you to get involved, or allows you to speak the word "Alzheimer's" with thoughtfulness and compassion, that's awesome. I would be satisfied with that. And my dad would be pleased. Thank you.

Part I

One Family's
Alzheimer's Journey

Thank You

Thank you for your curiosity about Alzheimer's disease. My father, Jack Moore, lived with this disease for about five years. During that time, my family took advantage of every resource available to us through the Alzheimer's Association. As a family living with Alzheimer's disease, those programs and services had a significant influence on our ability to care for our dad.

I know I don't stand here alone. I know everyone has a story. Statistically, it's likely that most people who hear about my family's situation have had or will have some connection with this devastating disease at some point. I appreciate the opportunity to share our version of the Alzheimer's story now.

A Perfect Family

First, let me tell you, I came from a perfect family. I am ninth of eleven children, raised in a regular, middle class household by regular, happy parents.

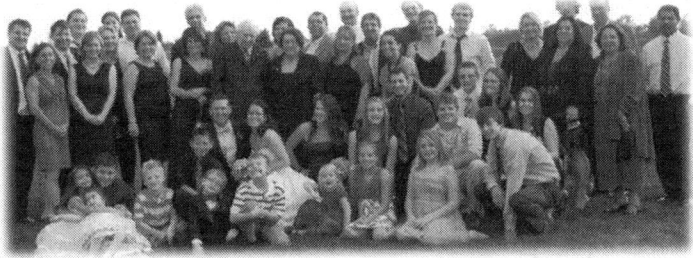

My dad would say he never worked a day in his life. He was born in Minneapolis, MN and, as a kid, rode the streetcar into town to watch the Millers games. He played catcher for the University of Minnesota. With the war on, opposing teams did not always have a catcher available, so dad would sometimes catch for both teams. Eventually, he went off to war along with the rest of his generation. After flying more than his requisite missions in the Pacific, he came home.

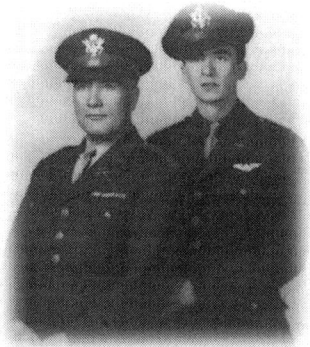

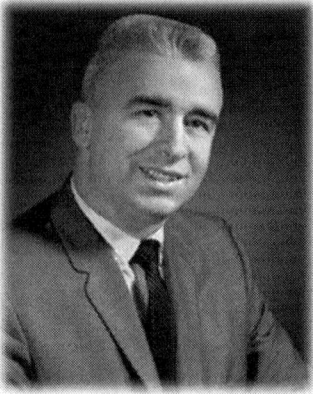

Dad went on to enjoy a long career in radio, which led him, eventually, to the Minnesota Broadcaster's Hall of Fame. In his free time, he was a president of the MNPGA, a major fundraiser for youth hockey, and for decades was a holder of season tickets to the Guthrie Theater in Minneapolis. I think the theater was my mom's idea.

More than anything, my dad enjoyed time with his family. We were lucky enough to have a little par three golf course behind our house and that was pretty much our playground every summer. Every one of us kids has memories of playing golf with our dad. He was the slowest putter.

After his kids had moved on to bigger and better golf courses, Dad volunteered as sort of a ranger for the youth golf league at the little course. He would sit in his folding chair along the sixth fairway and tell kids where their bad shots landed. Some of those shots hit him in the head on their way to landing in the woods, but he always laughed when he talked about that. He just loved that game.

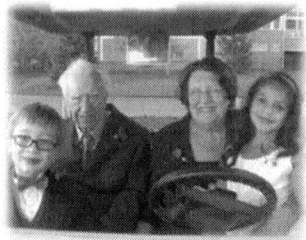

Dementia Can Sneak Up On You

When Dad was 80 years old, he endured a triple by-pass on what had long been a perfectly healthy heart. When he was 84, he encountered more heart trouble, but was still so remarkably healthy otherwise that his doctors hooked him up with a pacemaker. When he was 85, he began to exhibit changes that we found hard to ignore.

Dementia can sneak up on you. I'm sure we missed a lot of the earliest signs. My siblings started comparing notes casually at first. Someone noticed that Dad was irritable, which was not usual for him; he was a lot of things, but he was not irritable, normally. Someone mentioned that dad had asked where the refrigerator was… while standing in front of the refrigerator. He could be carrying on a perfectly normal dinner conversation and then look down at his fork and ask, "What's this for?"

We were slow to notice, I think, because, in many ways Dad was still himself. He was writing a book during this time, which, cognitively, can be a complex activity. Yet, he would call me two or three times a week to ask how to turn off the caps lock key on his computer. I know I didn't wish to see a bigger problem. I put a red X on the caps lock key so he would avoid it, and then I removed that key altogether.

This was about when that my mom revealed that she had been helping dad to get dressed.

"You mean, you pick out his sweater and tie?" I asked.

"No, I tell him the shirt goes over his head and the socks go on his feet."

Dad received his first guitar when he was sixteen years old. He played in bands through his 20's and continued to enjoy playing until just weeks before his death.

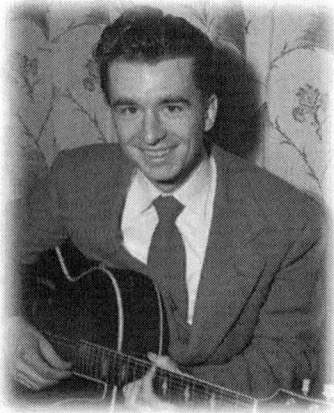

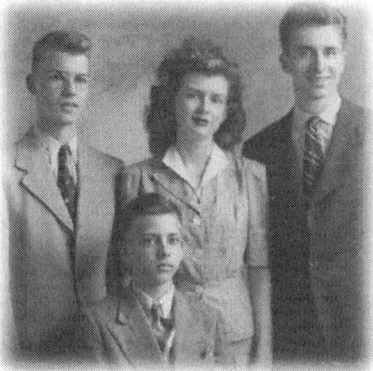

Does dementia run in families? Along with age, family history and genetics are leading risk factors for developing Alzheimer's Disease. Three out of the four siblings in Dad's family have been diagnosed.

Getting a Diagnosis

Some people ask if it was hard to get an Alzheimer's diagnosis. We were different from other families, perhaps, because, to be honest, we did not want an Alzheimer's diagnosis. My dad, himself, did not think he was ill. Our focus was not so much, "What's wrong?" as it was, "How can we make things easier?"

To complicate the situation, Dad was always on his A-game with the doctors, so even they could be fooled. After my father told his wife of fifty-plus years to leave because he did not want a stranger in the house, we approached the internist who had cared for dad for years; they were friends, I would say.

We explained what was going on and asked for an assessment. The doctor agreed, reluctantly, telling us he did not expect to find anything interesting. A nurse sat down with my dad and asked him a series of questions. This is how his Alzheimer's disease was diagnosed. She asked him to fold a piece of paper. She asked the political junky for the name of the President. She asked this man who had always been very casual about time to draw a picture of a clock. There were, maybe, twenty or twenty-five questions. My dad did not get a single right answer.

An Alzheimer's diagnosis brings with it some cultural stigma due to ignorance of the disease. Even my dad, if he heard us talking about it, would say, "There's nothing wrong with me." And in many ways, there wasn't anything wrong with him. He was still a wise man. He still had a sharp mind. He could still drive a golf ball as well as anybody his age. AND he had Alzheimer's disease.

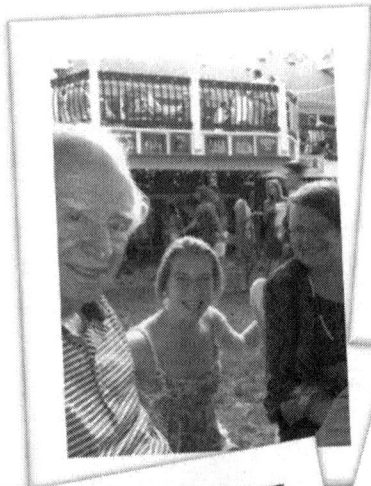

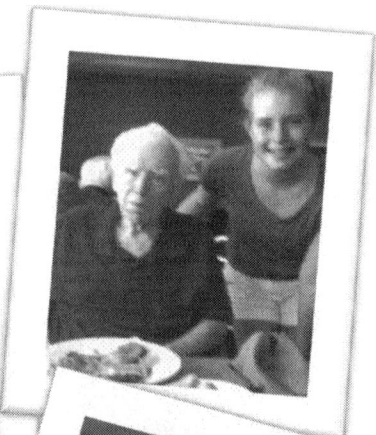

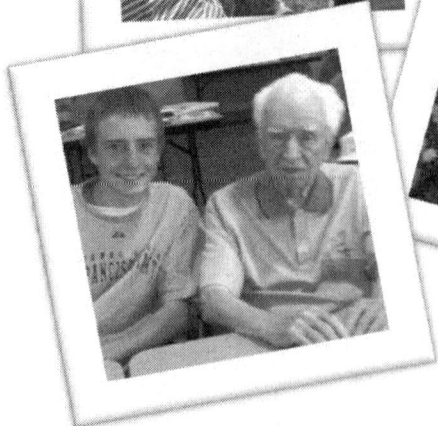

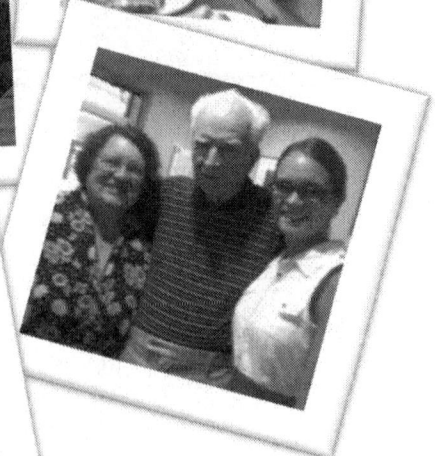

Isolation, Frustration & Hope

Families living with Alzheimer's disease can feel pretty isolated. We kind of thought, no one who hasn't been through this, you know – been there, done that – can really understand what it's like. And we had so many questions: What does this diagnosis even mean? What will our future look like? How quickly will this disease affect our dad? What can we do to help?

We called a family friend who works with seniors in St. Paul, MN, who suggested we get in touch with the Alzheimer's Association. It was somewhere to start. What we did not know at the time was that this would be the single most impactful phone call we would make.

Through the Alzheimer's Association, we discovered a whole community of people who understand the complex challenges of living as a family with this disease. We were able to replace isolation and frustration with hope and patience and coping skills.

The team at the Alzheimer's Association showed us charts and diagrams about the disease and described the changes we could expect to see as the disease progressed. In hindsight, I wonder if they have offices in Las Vegas – their predictions were uncannily accurate.

They explained the various treatment options that would be available to our dad. They knew about the latest breakthroughs in Alzheimer's research and they knew how long each medication or therapy might be effective.

They also provided us with the language we needed to communicate effectively with dad's primary care physician so dad could get what he needed there. In the end, that doctor thanked us. He told us he learned a lot from treating my dad.

To date, there is no cure for Alzheimer's disease. There is no way to stop or even slow the progression of the disease. There is no way to prevent it. There are, however, some treatment options that make life more livable on a day-to-day basis.

Dad was always creative, but he was never crafty. Working alongside an Art Therapist trained to help those with dementia and Alzheimer's disease, Dad took up painting for the first time in his life. Painting gave Dad an opportunity to follow instructions, to communicate with people, and to realize that sense of accomplishment that we all need to feel once in a while. He called this one, "Airplane Blues." It was framed and on exhibit, along with several others, in the foyer of his building.

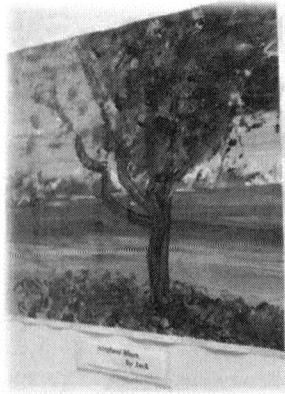

Care for the Caregivers

Our contacts at the Alzheimer's Association invited our family to participate in a pilot caregiving program. If I remember correctly, the criteria for getting into the caregiver's program were pretty simple: I think we needed to have a family member with a doctor's diagnosis of Alzheimer's disease and we had to demonstrate family participation in caregiving. We were offered one-on-one support sessions for my mother and group meetings for the whole family. We are not a group meeting sort of group, but we all went, anyway. We sort of looked at this as a learning opportunity. And it was something we could "do."

When we arrived for our first meeting at the Alzheimer's Association's office, my family pretty much filled up the waiting room. Remember, there are a lot of us. But no one there seemed to mind. They whisked us into a meeting room and cheerfully set up the phones so our out-of-town siblings could participate. Our Association Care Consultant was our fearless leader during these sessions. She was both incredibly patient and incredibly resourceful.

The meetings were all well organized and we never knew quite what to expect. At one meeting, we arrived to find the table in our conference room covered with picture cards. We were told to walk around and choose two cards: one representing our relationship with our father before Alzheimer's disease, and one representing our relationship with him now.

Our out-of-town siblings (on conference call) were instructed to peruse the objects in the room around them and choose two objects in the same way. Then we took turns explaining our selections.

My brother chose a single card: a picture of a man's hand holding a tiny new bird. He explained, "Before Alzheimer's, Dad carried me and protected me. Now, it's my turn to do the same thing for him." Just having a forum for putting feelings like that into words was so awesome.

There came a time when we knew our parents had to move into some kind of assisted living facility. Their home meant the world to our parents, but we felt like, for their safety, and especially for our mother's well-being, they had no choice but to move. Our town has many options for assisted living and memory care, so touring facilities was something of an ongoing family event and we broached this subject with our Care Consultant during one of those family meetings.

Our consultant suggested that we might have another option. She explained that, if we fully utilized the Association's programs and resources, our parents could probably stay in their own home safely and comfortably for another year and a half. What I want to tell you is that, when our parents did end up moving, it was a full eighteen months later.

Stage Six

From the Alzheimer's Association's website, we learned that Alzheimer's disease comes in seven stages, and some of those stages overlap. Stage Six indicates that the disease is pretty far along; it is marked by severe cognitive decline. At Stage Six, a person requires extensive help with daily activities because he (or she) loses track of who he is and whom he is with. A person in Stage Six might put his shoes on the wrong feet, and carrying on a conversation becomes really tough. But even at Stage Six, Alzheimer's disease had its surprising moments for our family.

I mentioned, my dad was a golfer. Even in Stage Six, when he could not do much for himself, Dad still liked to go out and hit a bucket of golf balls once in a while. One afternoon during Dad's last summer, my sister took him to the driving range. But it was much too hot for him and she parked way too far away. To make it worse, she accidentally bought a big bucket of balls instead of a small one.

She said it was awful. Dad was frustrated but determined to make the most of every one of the balls in that bucket. My sister described scrambling around behind Dad, hitting balls as fast as she could to get rid of them, while alternately pointing him in the right direction and encouraging him with all the lines he used to use with us, "We're here to have fun!" and, "It's a beautiful day!" and, "Keep your eye on the ball!"

When Dad and his clubs and my exhausted sister were finally back in the car, Dad turned to her and said, "I was really cutting it up out there, and you helped me. Thank you." Because of who Dad was, we knew we had to get past our frustrations and stay focused on finding solutions.

Through Alzheimer's disease, we learned how to live in the moment, how to find joy, and how to get creative about keeping Dad engaged and connected every day. We benefitted tremendously from the Alzheimer's Association's resources and we were constantly reminded of the value of our most important resource: each other.

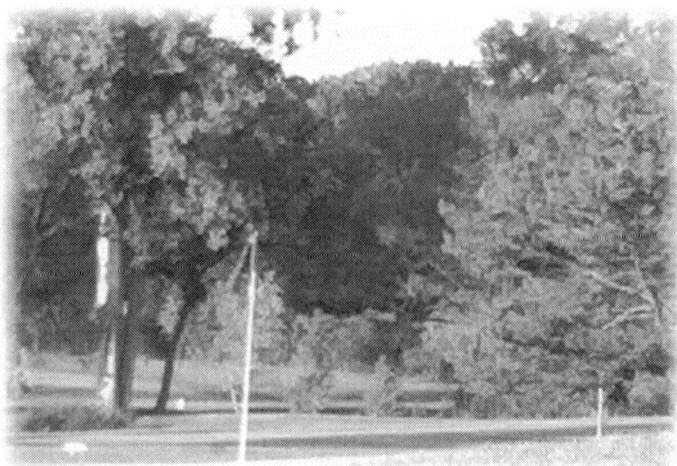

I Am Satisfied

My dad lived with Alzheimer's disease for almost five years. My family is grateful for the support we received from many extraordinary people during his illness. But we hope other families will have a story with a different ending.

Dad did not die from Alzheimer's. He died with Alzheimer's disease after a brief battle with cancer, one week shy of his 90th birthday.

Just before he passed, more clearly than he had asked for breakfast or anything for a long time, my father said two things.

He said, "I am satisfied."

And he said, "Protect families."

I can think of no better way to protect families than to find an end to Alzheimer's disease.

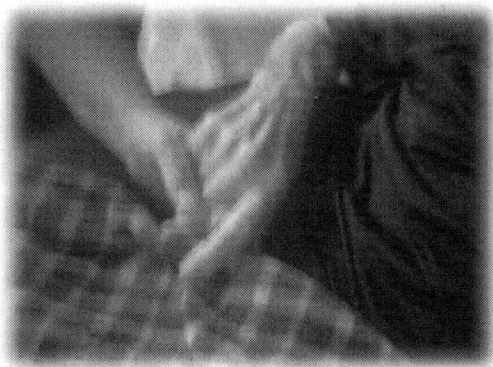

Part II

Walk to End
Alzheimer's Disease

Chela's
Personal Narrative

A little history:

Grasiela (we call her Chela) Hernandez loved her Grandpa. And that's an understatement. Chela is one of my dad's more than thirty grandchildren. She spent most of her preschool years living about a mile from my parents, and she regularly spent long days there with them.

Together, Chela and her grandparents played board games and worked out on the Wii; they hit golf balls, made cookies, read books, and prayed before meals. Chela's a happy, creative, caring kid by nature, and she brought a lot of joy to my parents during those years.

Shortly after she became tied up in the business of kindergarten, her grandparents moved away from their big red house; the sprawling summer days together became quick visits between dance lessons, birthday parties, homework and all the other demands a kid has on her time in those important elementary school years.

As a third grader, Chela participated, with our family, in the Walk to End Alzheimer's Disease. A few months after that, she was asked to write a personal narrative, which she did. She selected the topic on her own, and excepting a couple typos, this is it, as she wrote it, her story about the time she walked for Alzheimer's…

The Time I Walked for Alzheimer's ☺

By Grasiela Hernandez

Can we go yet??? I wanted to go to Target Field for an Alzheimer's walk☺ Soon enough we left!

My whole family was there! First we had to sign in and get our new t-shirts! They said "Jack's Blue Jays!' My cousin thought of the name.

I donated all of my money and everyone clapped for me! Oh boy did that feel good! Even when I only had change!!! Now I have a box that I'm going to fill up with change then at a machine I will cash it in for money and turn it in next year!!!

Next we sat down in the front row because we were the honorary family!!! There were 6,000 people there!!! My aunt gave a speech in front of all 6,000 people. ☺ She talked about my grandpa and how we reacted when we found out he had Alzheimer's disease. She did GREAT!!!

We also got flowers! There were different colors depending on which thing happened to you. Our family got purple flowers because we had a family member who passed from Alzheimer's ☹ ☹ ☹ They blew in the wind! I even gave one to my friend, Lexi.T!!!

I also got a sticker that said "WALK TO THE END OF ALZHEIMER'S!" It was purple!!

Soon it was time to walk!! Both of my grandmas didn't walk ☹ They just waited, but the rest of the family did walk☺ We could have walked 1 or 3 miles. I only walked 1 mile. Same with the rest of the family! I remember crossing the finish line! They clapped like crazy and cheered all around! It was awesome and I had fun!

After the walk, my family went out to eat. That was a lot of fun too ☺ I ate a cheeseburger with no pickles and then I also wanted a Coke but they gave me a Pepsi. Which was fine, but you know. I got to see my baby cousin Dylan! He is a one year old cutie pie!

Well after that we gave my grandma a ride home! She lives kind of far☹ I had a lot of fun and I can't wait to go next year!!! Now do you want to go, too?
If you do, save up ☺

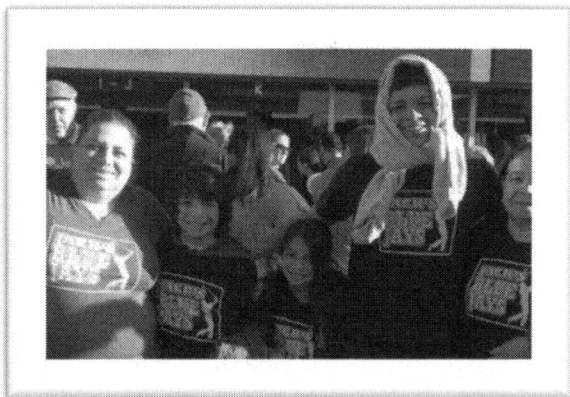

Thanks Again

Thank you for picking up this book and for taking a moment to be a part of our story. If you would like more information and additional resources, please check in with your local chapter of the Alzheimer's Association, www.alz.org.

This book is about one family's experience. It mentions the Alzheimer's Association, but it was not commissioned, sponsored nor supported by them However, proceeds from this book will be donated, in part, to the Association, in the interest of finding a way to end Alzheimer's disease.

If you feel compelled to take action against Alzheimer's, there are many ways to do so. You might be in a position to work on efforts to prevent or cure this disease. You might choose to assist financially, or you might choose to volunteer your time to help someone who is caring for someone with Alzheimer's disease. Maybe you'll make dinner for a caregiver. Maybe you will have an extra dose of patience when you're in the checkout line and the person ahead of you is confused or moving slowly. Maybe you'll send up a thought to the heavens for those living with Alzheimer's now. Whatever you can do, it is enough, and it helps.

It's all about families. Protect families. Thank you.

75426510R00020

Made in the USA
San Bernardino, CA
29 April 2018